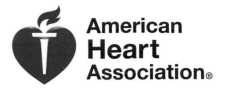

American
Heart
Association®

BLS for Healthcare Providers

STUDENT MANUAL

Editor

Mary Fran Hazinski, RN, MSN, *Senior Science Editor*

Senior Managing Editor

S. Lynn Hunter-Wilson

Special Contributors

Janet Butler, MS, *BLS HCP Writer*
Robin R. Hemphill, MD, MPH, *Content Consultant*
Robert A. Berg, MD
Diana M. Cave, RN, MSN
Marc D. Berg, MD
Diana D. Elmore, RN
Michael R. Sayre, MD
Peter A. Meaney, MD, MPH
Louis Gonzales, BS, LP
David Rogers, EdS, NREMT-P

BLS Subcommittee 2010-2011

Robert A. Berg, MD, *Chair*
Diana M. Cave, RN, MSN, *Immediate Past Chair, 2007-2009*
Ben Bobrow, MD
Carolyn L. Cason, RN, PhD
Paul S. Chan, MD, MSc
Todd J. Crocco, MD
Michael Cudnik, MD, MPH
Mohamud Daya, MD, MS
Dana P. Edelson, MD, MS
Barbara Furry, RNC, MS, CCRN
Raúl J. Gazmuri, MD, PhD
Theresa Hoadley, RN, PhD, TNS
Elizabeth A. Hunt, MD, MPH
Victor Johnson, EMT-P
Mary Beth Mancini, RN, PhD
Peter A. Meaney, MD, MPH
James Newcome, NREMT-P
Thomas D. Rea, MD, MPH
Robert Swor, DO
Andrew H. Travers, MD, MSc
Brian Walsh, RRT

© 2011 American Heart Association
ISBN 978-1-61669-039-7
Printed in the United States of America

First American Heart Association Printing March 2011
15 14 13 12 11 10 9 8 7 6 5 4 3 2 1

i

To find out about any updates or corrections to this text, visit **www.heart.org/cpr**, navigate to the page for this course, and click on "Updates."

Contents

Part 8
Mouth-to-Mouth Breaths

Part 9
Rescue Breathing

Part 10
Relief of Choking

Appendix

Recommended Reading

Part 1

General Concepts

Introduction

Welcome to the BLS for Healthcare Providers Course. With the knowledge and skills you learn in this course, you can save a life. You will learn the skills of CPR for victims of all ages and will practice CPR in a team setting. You will learn how to use an automated external defibrillator (AED) and how to relieve choking (foreign-body airway obstruction). The skills you learn in this course will enable you to recognize emergencies such as sudden cardiac arrest and know how to respond to them.

Despite important advances in prevention, cardiac arrest remains a substantial public health problem and a leading cause of death in many parts of the world. Cardiac arrest occurs both in and out of the hospital. In the United States and Canada, approximately 350 000 people per year (approximately half of them in-hospital) have a cardiac arrest and receive attempted resuscitation. This estimate does not include the substantial number of victims who have an arrest without attempted resuscitation.

The Purpose of This Manual

This manual focuses on what healthcare providers need to know to perform CPR in a wide variety of in- and out-of-hospital settings. The manual details the information and skills you will learn in this class:

- Initiating the Chain of Survival
- Performing prompt, high-quality chest compressions for adult, child, and infant victims
- Initiating early use of an AED
- Providing appropriate rescue breaths
- Practicing 2-rescuer team CPR
- Relieving choking

> **Critical Concepts**
>
> High-quality CPR improves a victim's chances of survival. The critical characteristics of high-quality CPR include
>
> - **Start compressions within 10 seconds** of recognition of cardiac arrest.
> - **Push hard, push fast:** Compress at a rate of at least 100/min with a depth of at least 2 inches (5 cm) for adults, approximately 2 inches (5 cm) for children, and approximately 1½ inches (4 cm) for infants.
> - **Allow complete chest recoil** after each compression.
> - **Minimize interruptions** in compressions (try to limit interruptions to <10 seconds).
> - **Give effective breaths** that make the chest rise.
> - **Avoid excessive ventilation.**

The Chain of Survival

Learning Objectives

After reading this section you will be able to name the links in the American Heart Association (AHA) adult Chain of Survival and state the importance of each link.

Introduction to the Adult Chain of Survival

The AHA has adopted, supported, and helped develop the concept of emergency cardiovascular care (ECC) systems for many years.

The term *Chain of Survival* provides a useful metaphor for the elements of the ECC systems concept (Figure 1). The 5 links in the adult Chain of Survival are

- Immediate **recognition** of cardiac arrest and **activation** of the emergency response system
- Early **cardiopulmonary resuscitation (CPR)** with an emphasis on chest compressions
- Rapid **defibrillation**
- Effective **advanced life support**
- Integrated **post–cardiac arrest care**

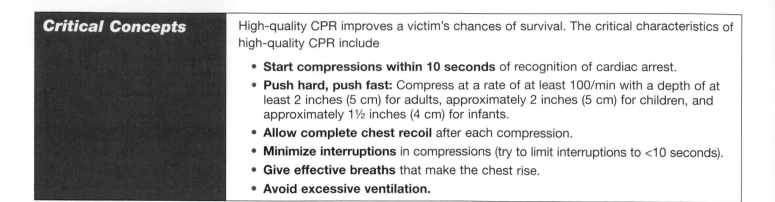

Figure 1. The adult Chain of Survival.

Although basic life support is taught as a sequence of distinct steps to enhance skills retention and clarify priorities, several actions should be accomplished **simultaneously** (eg, begin CPR and activate the emergency response system) when multiple rescuers are present.

Introduction to the Pediatric Chain of Survival

Although in adults cardiac arrest is often sudden and results from a cardiac cause, in children cardiac arrest is often secondary to respiratory failure and shock. Identifying children with these problems is essential to reduce the likelihood of pediatric cardiac arrest and maximize survival and recovery. Therefore, a prevention link is added in the pediatric Chain of Survival (Figure 2):

- **Prevention** of arrest
- Early high-quality **bystander CPR**
- Rapid **activation** of the EMS (or other emergency response) system
- Effective **advanced life support** (including rapid stabilization and transport to definitive care and rehabilitation)
- Integrated **post–cardiac arrest care**

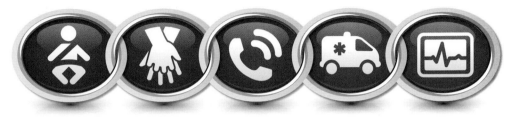

Figure 2. The pediatric Chain of Survival.

2010 AHA Guidelines for CPR and ECC Science Update

Overview

The *2010 American Heart Association Guidelines for Cardiopulmonary Resuscitation and Emergency Cardiovascular Care* recommendations for healthcare providers include the following key changes and issues:

- Changes in basic life support (BLS) sequence
- Continued emphasis on high-quality CPR, with minor changes in compression rate and depth
- Additional changes regarding cricoid pressure, pulse check, and AED use in infants

Learning Objectives

After reading this section you will be able to name the major science updates in the *2010 AHA Guidelines for CPR and ECC.*

Change in Sequence: C-A-B, Not A-B-C

The *2010 AHA Guidelines for CPR and ECC* recommend a change in the BLS sequence of steps from A-B-C (Airway, Breathing, Chest compressions) to C-A-B (Chest compressions, Airway, Breathing) for adults, children, and infants. This change in CPR sequence requires reeducation of everyone who has ever learned CPR, but the consensus of the authors and experts involved in creating the *2010 AHA Guidelines for CPR and ECC* is that the change is likely to improve survival.

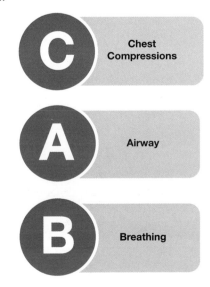

In the A-B-C sequence, chest compressions were often delayed while the rescuer opened the airway to give mouth-to-mouth breaths, retrieved a barrier device, or gathered and assembled ventilation equipment. By changing the sequence to C-A-B, rescuers can start chest compressions sooner, and the delay in giving breaths should be minimal (only the time required to deliver the first cycle of 30 chest compressions, or approximately 18 seconds or less; for 2-rescuer infant or child CPR, the delay will be even shorter).

Emphasis on High-Quality CPR

The *2010 AHA Guidelines for CPR and ECC* once again emphasize the need for high-quality CPR, including

- A compression rate of at least 100/min (this is a change from "approximately" 100/min).
- A compression depth of at least 2 inches (5 cm) in adults and a compression depth of at least one third of the anterior-posterior diameter of the chest in infants and children. This is approximately 1½ inches (4 cm) in infants and 2 inches (5 cm) in children. Note that the range of 1½ to 2 inches is no longer used for adults, and the absolute depth specified for children and infants is deeper than in previous versions of the *AHA Guidelines for CPR and ECC*.
- Allowing complete chest recoil, minimizing interruptions in compressions, and avoiding excessive ventilation continue to be important components of high-quality CPR.

To further strengthen the focus on high-quality CPR, the *2010 AHA Guidelines for CPR and ECC* stress the importance of training using a team approach to CPR. The steps in the BLS Algorithm have traditionally been presented as a sequence to help a single rescuer prioritize actions.

There is increased focus on providing CPR as a team because resuscitations in most EMS and healthcare systems involve teams of rescuers, with rescuers performing several actions simultaneously. For example, one rescuer activates the emergency response system while a second begins chest compressions, a third is either providing ventilations or retrieving the bag-mask for rescue breathing, and a fourth is retrieving a defibrillator and preparing to use it.

No Look, Listen, and Feel

Another key change is the removal of "look, listen, and feel for breathing" from the assessment step. This step was removed because bystanders often failed to start CPR when they observed agonal gasping. The healthcare provider should not delay activating the emergency response system but should check the victim for 2 things simultaneously: response and breathing. With the new chest compression–first sequence, the rescuer should activate the emergency response system and begin CPR if the adult victim is unresponsive and not breathing or not breathing normally (only gasping) and has no pulse. For the child or infant victim, CPR is performed if the victim is unresponsive and not breathing or only gasping and has no pulse.

For victims of all ages (except newborns), begin CPR with compressions (C-A-B sequence). After each set of chest compressions, open the airway and give 2 breaths.

Additional Changes

There are several additional changes in the *2010 AHA Guidelines for CPR and ECC*:

Change	Details
The routine use of cricoid pressure in cardiac arrest is not recommended	Although cricoid pressure can prevent gastric inflation and reduce the risk of regurgitation and aspiration during bag-mask ventilation, it may also block ventilation.
	Several randomized studies have shown that cricoid pressure can delay or prevent the placement of an advanced airway and that some aspiration can still occur despite the use of cricoid pressure. In addition, it is difficult to appropriately train rescuers how to do this.
	Therefore, the routine use of cricoid pressure in cardiac arrest is not recommended.
Continued de-emphasis of the pulse check	It can be difficult to determine the presence or absence of a pulse within 10 seconds, especially in an emergency, and studies show that both healthcare providers and lay rescuers are unable to reliably detect a pulse.
	If the victim is unresponsive and not breathing or only gasping, healthcare providers may take up to 10 seconds to attempt to feel for a pulse (brachial in an infant and carotid or femoral in a child).
	If within 10 seconds you don't feel a pulse or are not sure if you feel a pulse, begin chest compressions.
Use of an AED for infants	For infants, a manual defibrillator is preferred to an AED for defibrillation.
	If a manual defibrillator is not available, an AED equipped with a pediatric dose attenuator is preferred.
	If neither is available, you may use an AED without a pediatric dose attenuator.

For more detailed information and references, read the *2010 AHA Guidelines for CPR and ECC,* including the Executive Summary, published online in *Circulation* in October 2010, or the *Highlights of the 2010 AHA Guidelines for CPR and ECC,* available at **www.heart.org/eccguidelines**. You can also review the detailed summary of resuscitation science in the *2010 International Consensus on Cardiopulmonary Resuscitation and Emergency Cardiovascular Care Science With Treatment Recommendations,* published simultaneously in *Circulation* and *Resuscitation*.

BLS/CPR for Adults

BLS/CPR Basics for Adults

Overview

This section describes the basic steps of CPR for adults. Adults include adolescents (ie, after the onset of puberty). Signs of puberty include chest or underarm hair in males and any breast development in females.

Learning Objectives

At the end of this section you will be able to

- Tell the basic steps of CPR for adults
- Show the basic steps of CPR for adults

Understanding the Basics of BLS

BLS consists of these main parts (Figure 3):

- **Chest compressions**
- **Airway**
- **Breathing**
- **Defibrillation**

You will learn about each of these throughout this course.

Distinct from the lone responder approach, many workplaces and most EMS and in-hospital resuscitations involve teams of providers who should perform several actions **simultaneously** (eg, one rescuer activates the emergency response system while a second rescuer begins chest compressions, a third is either providing ventilations or retrieving the bag-mask for rescue breathing, and a fourth is retrieving a defibrillator and preparing to use it). This course focuses on team-based CPR.

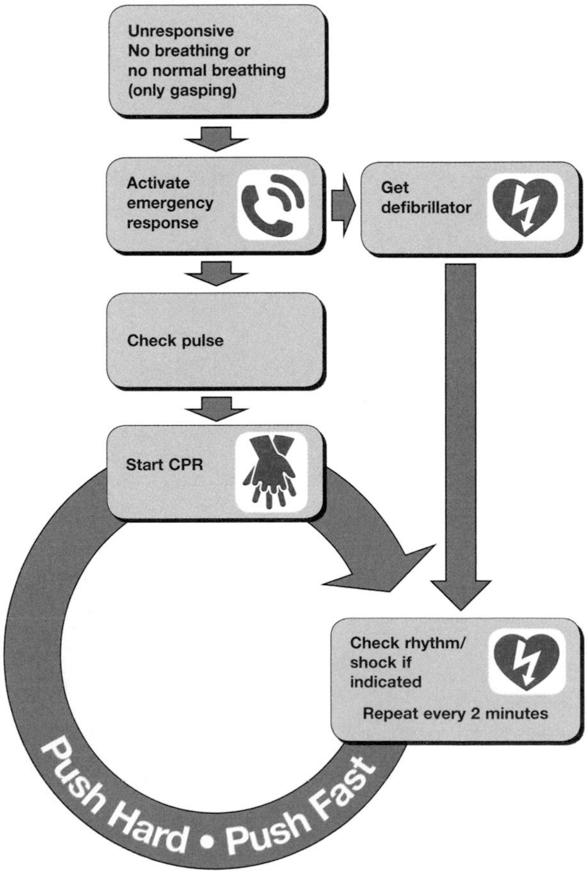

Figure 3. The Simplified Adult BLS Algorithm for **Healthcare Providers**.

Overview of Initial BLS Steps

Follow these initial BLS steps for adults:

Step	Action
1	**Assess** the victim for a response and look for normal or abnormal breathing. If there is no response and no breathing or no normal breathing (ie, only gasping), shout for help.
2	If you are alone, **activate the emergency response system** and get an AED (or defibrillator) if available and return to the victim.
3	Check the victim's **pulse** (take at least 5 but no more than 10 seconds).
4	If you do not definitely feel a pulse within 10 seconds, **perform 5 cycles of compressions and breaths** (30:2 ratio), starting with compressions (C-A-B sequence).

Step 1: Assessment and Scene Safety

The first rescuer who arrives at the side of the victim must quickly be sure that the scene is safe. The rescuer should then check the victim for a response:

Step	Action
1	Make sure the scene is safe for you and the victim. You do not want to become a victim yourself.
2	Tap the victim's shoulder and shout, "Are you all right?" (Figure 4).
3	Check to see if the victim is breathing. If a victim is not breathing or not breathing normally (ie, only gasping), you must activate the emergency response system.

Caution
Agonal Gasps

Agonal gasps are not normal breathing. Agonal gasps may be present in the first minutes after sudden cardiac arrest.

A person who gasps usually looks like he is drawing air in very quickly. The mouth may be open and the jaw, head, or neck may move with gasps. Gasps may appear forceful or weak, and some time may pass between gasps because they usually happen at a slow rate. The gasp may sound like a snort, snore, or groan. Gasping is not normal breathing. It is a sign of cardiac arrest in someone who doesn't respond.

If a victim is not breathing or there is no normal breathing (ie, only agonal gasps), you must activate the emergency response system, check the pulse, and start CPR.

Step 2: Activate the Emergency Response System and Get an AED

If you are alone and find an unresponsive victim not breathing, shout for help. If no one responds, activate the emergency response system, get an AED (or defibrillator) if available, and then return to the victim to check a pulse and begin CPR (C-A-B sequence).

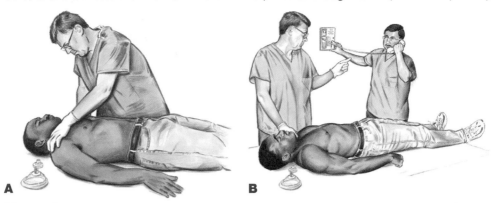

Figure 4. Check for response and breathing and activate the emergency response system (assess and activate). **A,** Tap the victim's shoulder and shout, "Are you all right?" At the same time, look for breathing. **B,** If the adult victim does not respond and has no breathing or no normal breathing (ie, is only gasping), shout for help. If another rescuer responds, send him or her to activate the emergency response system and get the AED (or defibrillator) if available. If no one responds, activate the emergency response system, get the AED (or defibrillator), and return to the victim to check a pulse and begin CPR (C-A-B sequence).

Step 3: Pulse Check

Healthcare providers should take no more than 10 seconds to check for a pulse.

Locating the Carotid Artery Pulse

To perform a pulse check in the adult, palpate a carotid pulse (Figure 5). If you do not definitely feel a pulse within 10 seconds, start chest compressions.

Follow these steps to locate the carotid artery pulse:

Step	Action
1	Locate the trachea, using 2 or 3 fingers (Figure 5A).
2	Slide these 2 or 3 fingers into the groove between the trachea and the muscles at the side of the neck, where you can feel the carotid pulse (Figure 5B).
3	Feel for a pulse *for at least 5 but no more than 10 seconds*. If you do not definitely feel a pulse, begin CPR, starting with chest compressions (C-A-B sequence).

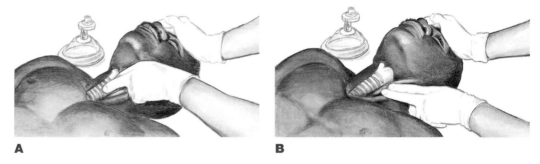

Figure 5. Finding the carotid pulse. **A,** Locate the trachea. **B,** Gently feel for the carotid pulse.

Step 4: Begin Cycles of 30 Chest Compressions and 2 Breaths (CPR)

The lone rescuer should use the compression-ventilation ratio of 30 compressions to 2 breaths when giving CPR to victims of any age.

When you give chest compressions, it is important to push the chest hard and fast, at a rate of at least 100 compressions per minute, allow the chest to recoil completely after each compression, and minimize interruptions in compressions. Begin with chest compressions.

Chest Compression Technique

The foundation of CPR is **chest compressions**. Follow these steps to perform chest compressions in an adult:

Step	Action
1	Position yourself at the victim's side.
2	Make sure the victim is lying faceup on a firm, flat surface. If the victim is lying facedown, carefully roll him faceup. If you suspect the victim has a head or neck injury, try to keep the head, neck, and torso in a line when rolling the victim to a faceup position.
3	Put the heel of one hand on the center of the victim's chest on the lower half of the breastbone (Figure 6A).
4	Put the heel of your other hand on top of the first hand.
5	Straighten your arms and position your shoulders directly over your hands.
6	**Push hard and fast.** • Press down at least 2 inches (5 cm) with each compression (this requires hard work). For each chest compression, make sure you push straight down on the victim's breastbone (Figure 6B). • Deliver compressions in a smooth fashion at a rate of **at least 100/min.**
7	At the end of each compression, make sure you allow the chest to recoil (re-expand) completely. Chest recoil allows blood to flow into the heart and is necessary for chest compressions to create blood flow. Incomplete chest recoil is harmful because it reduces the blood flow created by chest compressions. Chest compression and chest recoil/relaxation times should be approximately equal.
8	Minimize interruptions.

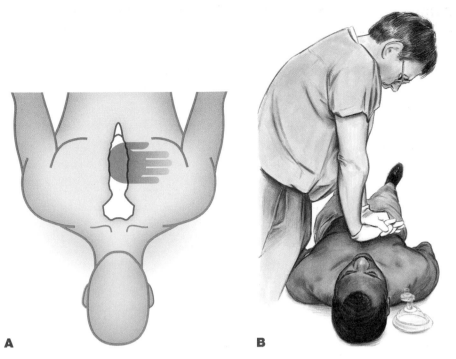

A   **B**

Figure 6. A, Place your hands on the breastbone in the center of the chest. **B,** Correct position of the rescuer during chest compressions.

Foundational Facts **The Importance of a Firm Surface**	Compressions pump the blood in the heart to the rest of the body. If a firm surface is under the victim, the force you use will be more likely to compress the chest and heart and create blood flow rather than simply push the victim into the mattress or other soft surface.

Foundational Facts **Alternate Technique for Chest Compressions**	If you have difficulty pushing deeply during compressions, put one hand on the breastbone to push on the chest. Grasp the wrist of that hand with your other hand to support the first hand as it pushes the chest (Figure 7). This technique is helpful for rescuers with arthritis. 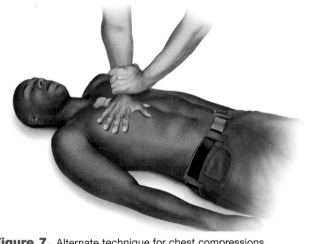 **Figure 7.** Alternate technique for chest compressions.

Moving the Victim Only When Necessary

Do not move the victim while CPR is in progress unless the victim is in a dangerous environment (such as a burning building) or if you believe you cannot perform CPR effectively in the victim's present position or location. CPR is better and has fewer interruptions when rescuers perform the resuscitation where they find the victim.

Opening the Airway for Breaths: Head Tilt–Chin Lift

There are 2 methods for opening the airway to provide breaths: head tilt–chin lift and jaw thrust. Two rescuers are generally needed to perform a jaw thrust and provide breaths with a bag-mask device. This is discussed in the "2-Rescuer Adult BLS/Team CPR Sequence" section. Use a jaw thrust only if you suspect a head or neck injury, as it may reduce neck and spine movement. Switch to a head tilt–chin lift maneuver if the jaw thrust does not open the airway.

Follow these steps to perform a head tilt–chin lift (Figure 8):

Step	Action
1	Place one hand on the victim's forehead and push with your palm to tilt the head back.
2	Place the fingers of the other hand under the bony part of the lower jaw near the chin.
3	Lift the jaw to bring the chin forward.

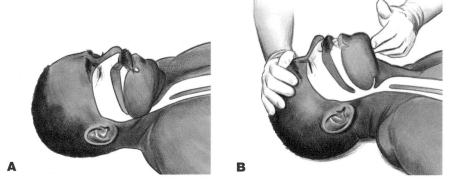

A **B**

Figure 8. The head tilt–chin lift relieves airway obstruction in an unresponsive victim. **A,** Obstruction by the tongue. When a victim is unresponsive, the tongue can block the upper airway. **B,** The head tilt–chin lift maneuver lifts the tongue, relieving airway obstruction.

Caution **Things to Avoid With Head Tilt–Chin Lift**	• Do not press deeply into the soft tissue under the chin because this might block the airway. • Do not use the thumb to lift the chin. • Do not close the victim's mouth completely.

Adult Mouth-to–Barrier Device Breathing

Standard precautions include using barrier devices, such as a face mask (Figure 9) or a bag-mask device, when giving breaths. Rescuers should replace face shields with mouth-to-mask or bag-mask devices at the first opportunity. Masks usually have a 1-way valve that diverts exhaled air, blood, or bodily fluids away from the rescuer.

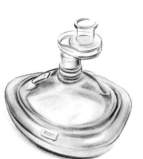

Figure 9. Face mask.

<table>
<tr><td>**Foundational Facts**
Low Infection Risk</td><td>The risk of infection from CPR is extremely low and limited to a few case reports, but the US Occupational Safety and Health Administration (OSHA) requires that healthcare workers use standard precautions in the workplace, including during CPR.</td></tr>
</table>

Giving Adult Mouth-to-Mask Breaths

For mouth-to-mask breaths, you use a mask with or without a 1-way valve. The 1-way valve allows the rescuer's breath to enter the victim's mouth and nose and diverts the victim's exhaled air away from the rescuer. Some masks have an oxygen inlet that allows you to administer supplementary oxygen.

Effective use of the mask barrier device requires instruction and supervised practice.

Giving Mouth-to-Mask Breaths

To use a mask, the lone rescuer is at the victim's side. This position is ideal when performing 1-rescuer CPR because you can give breaths and perform chest compressions when positioned at the victim's side. The lone rescuer holds the mask against the victim's face and opens the airway with a head tilt–chin lift.

Follow these steps to open the airway with a head tilt–chin lift and use a mask to give breaths to the victim:

Step	Action
1	Position yourself at the victim's side.
2	Place the mask on the victim's face, using the bridge of the nose as a guide for correct position.
3	Seal the mask against the face: • Using the hand that is closer to the top of the victim's head, place your index finger and thumb along the edge of the mask. • Place the thumb of your second hand along the bottom edge of the mask.
4	Place the remaining fingers of your second hand along the bony margin of the jaw and lift the jaw. Perform a head tilt–chin lift to open the airway (Figure 10).
5	While you lift the jaw, press firmly and completely around the outside edge of the mask to seal the mask against the face.
6	Deliver air over 1 second to make the victim's chest rise.

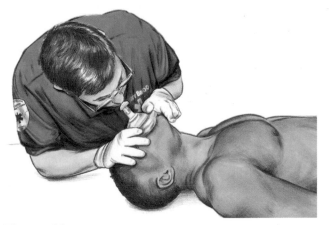

Figure 10. Mouth-to-mask breaths, 1 rescuer. The rescuer performs 1-rescuer CPR from a position at the victim's side. Perform a head tilt–chin lift to open the airway while holding the mask tightly against the face.

Bag-Mask Device

Bag-mask devices consist of a bag attached to a face mask. They may also include a 1-way valve. Bag-mask devices are the most common method that healthcare providers use to give positive-pressure ventilation during CPR. The bag-mask ventilation technique requires instruction and practice and is not recommended by a lone rescuer during CPR.

Using the Bag-Mask During 2-Rescuer CPR

Follow these steps to open the airway with a head tilt–chin lift and use a bag-mask to give breaths to the victim:

Step	Action
1	Position yourself directly above the victim's head.
2	Place the mask on the victim's face, using the bridge of the nose as a guide for correct position.
3	Use the E-C clamp technique to hold the mask in place while you lift the jaw to hold the airway open (Figure 11): • Perform a head tilt. • Place the mask on the face with the narrow portion at the bridge of the nose. • Use the thumb and index finger of one hand to make a "C" on the side of the mask, pressing the edges of the mask to the face. • Use the remaining fingers to lift the angles of the jaw (3 fingers form an "E"), open the airway, and press the face to the mask.
4	Squeeze the bag to give breaths (1 second each) while watching for chest rise. Deliver all breaths over 1 second whether or not you use supplementary oxygen.

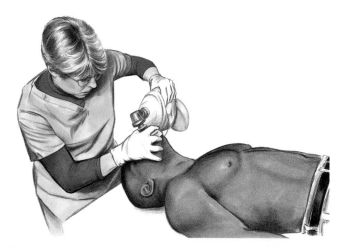

Figure 11. Mouth-to-mask E-C clamp technique of holding mask while lifting the jaw. Position yourself at the victim's head. Place the thumb and first finger around the top of the mask (forming a "C") while using the third, fourth, and fifth fingers (forming an "E") to lift the jaw.

Foundational Facts

Giving Breaths With Supplementary Oxygen

If you are using supplementary oxygen with a bag-mask device, you will still deliver each breath over 1 second. If you use only 1 second per breath for any method of delivery, you can help minimize the interruptions in chest compressions needed for breaths and avoid excessive ventilation.

2-Rescuer Adult BLS/Team CPR Sequence

Overview

This section explains how to perform 2-rescuer team CPR for adults.

Learning Objectives

At the end of this section you will be able to show how to perform 2-rescuer team CPR.

When More Rescuers Arrive

When a second rescuer is available to help, that second rescuer should activate the emergency response system and get the AED. The first rescuer should remain with the victim to start CPR immediately, beginning with chest compressions. After the second rescuer returns, the rescuers should use the AED as soon as it is available. The rescuers will then give compressions and breaths but should switch roles after every 5 cycles of CPR (about every 2 minutes).

As additional rescuers arrive, they can help with the bag-mask ventilation, use of the AED or defibrillator, and crash cart.

Duties for Each Rescuer

In 2-rescuer CPR (Figure 12), each rescuer has specific duties:

Rescuer	Location	Duties
Rescuer 1	At the victim's side	• Perform chest compressions. – Compress the chest at least 2 inches (5 cm). – Compress at a rate of at least 100/min. – Allow the chest to recoil completely after each compression. – Minimize interruptions in compressions (try to limit any interruptions in chest compressions to <10 seconds). – Use a compressions-to-breaths ratio of 30:2. – Count compressions aloud. • Switch duties with the second rescuer every 5 cycles or about 2 minutes, taking <5 seconds to switch.
Rescuer 2	At the victim's head	• Maintain an open airway using either – Head tilt–chin lift – Jaw thrust • Give breaths, watching for chest rise and avoiding excessive ventilation. • Encourage the first rescuer to perform compressions that are deep enough and fast enough and to allow complete chest recoil between compressions. • Switch duties with the first rescuer every 5 cycles or about 2 minutes, taking <5 seconds to switch.

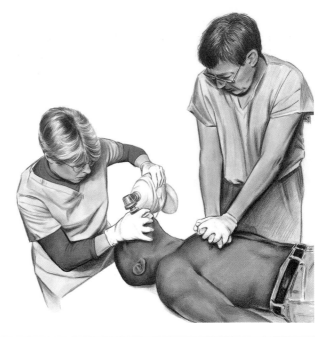

Figure 12. Two-rescuer CPR. The first rescuer performs chest compressions. The second rescuer performs bag-mask ventilation using a mask with supplementary oxygen (when available). The second rescuer ensures that the chest rises with each breath. Rescuers should switch roles after 5 cycles of CPR (about every 2 minutes).

| **Foundational Facts**

Effective Team Performance to Minimize Interruptions in Compressions | Effective teams communicate continuously. If the compressor counts out loud, the rescuer providing breaths can anticipate when breaths will be given and prepare to give them efficiently to minimize interruptions in compressions. The count will also help both rescuers to know when the time for a switch is approaching.

It is hard work to deliver effective chest compressions. If the compressor tires, chest compressions won't be as effective. To reduce rescuer fatigue, switch compressor roles every 5 cycles (about 2 minutes). To minimize interruptions, perform the switch when the AED is analyzing the rhythm and take no more than 5 seconds to switch. |

2 Rescuers Using the Bag-Mask

When 3 or more rescuers are present, 2 rescuers can provide more effective bag-mask ventilation than 1 rescuer. When 2 rescuers use the bag-mask system, one rescuer opens the airway with a head tilt–chin lift (or jaw thrust) and holds the mask to the face while the other rescuer squeezes the bag (Figure 13). All professional rescuers should learn both the 1- and 2-rescuer bag-mask ventilation techniques. When possible in the course, practice with devices for both bag-mask and mouth-to-mask ventilation.

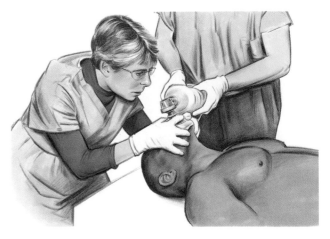

Figure 13. Two-rescuer bag-mask ventilation. The rescuer at the victim's head tilts the victim's head and seals the mask against the victim's face with the thumb and first finger of each hand, creating a "C" to provide a complete seal around the edges of the mask. The rescuer uses the remaining 3 fingers (the "E") to lift the jaw (this holds the airway open) and hold the face up against the mask. The second rescuer slowly squeezes the bag (over 1 second) until the chest rises. Both rescuers should watch for chest rise.

Opening the Airway for Breaths: Jaw Thrust

If the victim has a head or neck injury and you suspect a spine injury, 2 rescuers may use another method to open the airway: a jaw thrust (Figure 14). Two people perform a jaw thrust while holding the neck still and giving bag-mask ventilation. If the jaw thrust does not open the airway, use a head tilt–chin lift.

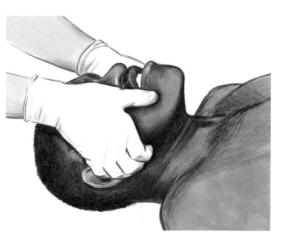

Figure 14. Jaw thrust without head tilt. The jaw is lifted without tilting the head. This is the airway maneuver of choice when the victim has a possible spine injury.

Follow these steps to perform a jaw thrust:

Step	Action
1	Place one hand on each side of the victim's head, resting your elbows on the surface on which the victim is lying.
2	Place your fingers under the angles of the victim's lower jaw and lift with both hands, displacing the jaw forward (Figure 14).
3	If the lips close, push the lower lip with your thumb to open the lips.

Automated External Defibrillator for Adults and Children 8 Years of Age and Older

Automated External Defibrillator for Adults and Children 8 Years of Age and Older

Overview

The interval from collapse to defibrillation is one of the most important determinants of survival from sudden cardiac arrest with ventricular fibrillation (see Foundational Facts, below) or pulseless ventricular tachycardia.

Automated external defibrillators (AEDs) are computerized devices that can identify cardiac rhythms that need a shock, and they can then deliver the shock. AEDs are simple to operate, allowing laypersons and healthcare providers to attempt defibrillation safely.

Learning Objectives

At the end of this section you will be able to

- List the steps common to the operation of all AEDs
- Show proper placement of the AED pads
- Recall when to press the SHOCK button when using an AED
- Explain why no one should touch the victim when prompted by the AED during analysis and shock delivery
- Describe the proper actions to take when the AED gives a "no shock indicated" (or "no shock advised") message
- Show coordination of CPR and AED use to minimize
    - Interruptions in chest compressions
    - Time between last compression and shock delivery
    - Time between shock delivery and resumption of chest compressions

AED Arrival

Once the AED arrives, place it at the victim's side, next to the rescuer who will operate it. This position provides ready access to the AED controls and easy placement of AED pads. It also allows a second rescuer to perform CPR from the opposite side of the victim without interfering with AED operation.

Note: If multiple rescuers are present, one rescuer should continue chest compressions while another rescuer attaches the AED pads.

Foundational Facts
Defibrillation

When ventricular fibrillation is present, the heart muscle fibers quiver and do not contract together to pump blood. A defibrillator delivers an electric shock to stop the quivering of the heart fibers. This allows the muscle fibers of the heart to "reset" so that they can begin to contract at the same time. Once an organized rhythm occurs, the heart muscle may begin to contract effectively and begin to generate a pulse (called return of spontaneous circulation, or ROSC).

AEDs are available in different models with a few differences from model to model, but all AEDs operate in basically the same way. There are 4 universal steps for operating an AED:

Note: To reduce the time to shock delivery, you should ideally be able to perform the first 2 steps within 30 seconds after the AED arrives at the victim's side.

Step	Action
1	**POWER ON the AED** (the AED will then guide you through the next steps). • Open the carrying case or the top of the AED. • Turn the power on (some devices will "power on" automatically when you open the lid or case).

2	**ATTACH** AED pads to the victim's bare chest.
	
	• Choose adult pads (not child pads or a child system) for victims 8 years of age and older.
	• Peel the backing away from the AED pads.
	• Attach the adhesive AED pads to the victim's bare chest.
	  – Place one AED pad on the victim's upper-right chest (directly below the collarbone).
	  – Place the other pad to the side of the left nipple, with the top edge of the pad a few inches below the armpit (Figure 15).
	• Attach the AED connecting cables to the AED box (some are preconnected).

3	"Clear" the victim and **ANALYZE** the rhythm. • If the AED prompts you, clear the victim during analysis. Be sure no one is touching the victim, not even the rescuer in charge of giving breaths. • Some AEDs will tell you to push a button to allow the AED to begin analyzing the heart rhythm; others will do that automatically. The AED may take about 5 to 15 seconds to analyze. • The AED then tells you if a shock is needed.
4	**If the AED advises a shock, it will tell you to clear the victim.** • Clear the victim before delivering the shock: be sure no one is touching the victim. • Loudly state a "clear the victim" message, such as "Everybody clear" or simply "Clear." • Look to be sure no one is in contact with the victim. • Press the **SHOCK** button. • The shock will produce a sudden contraction of the victim's muscles.
5	If no shock is needed, and after any shock delivery, **immediately resume CPR,** starting with chest compressions.
6	After 5 cycles or about 2 minutes of CPR, the AED will prompt you to repeat steps 3 and 4. If "no shock advised," immediately restart CPR beginning with chest compressions.

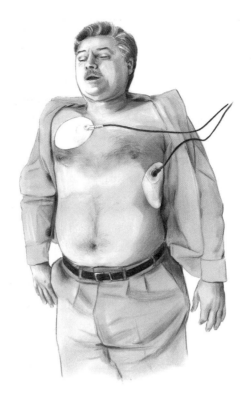

Figure 15. AED pad placement on the victim.

Foundational Facts **Importance of Minimizing Time Between Last Compression and Shock Delivery**	Analysis of thousands of rhythm strips recorded before and after shock delivery has shown that if rescuers can keep the time between the last compression and shock delivery to 10 seconds or less, the shock is much more likely to be effective (ie, to eliminate ventricular fibrillation and result in return of spontaneous circulation). Effectiveness of shock delivery decreases significantly for every additional 10 seconds that elapses between last compression and shock delivery. Minimizing this interval will require practice and excellent team coordination, particularly between the compressor and the rescuer operating the defibrillator.

Caution **Moving the Victim**	You may leave an AED attached while transporting the victim on a stretcher or in an ambulance. Never push the ANALYZE button while moving the victim. Because movement can interfere with rhythm analysis and artifacts can simulate ventricular fibrillation, the rescuer must bring the stretcher or vehicle to a complete stop and then reanalyze.

Special Situations

The following special situations may require the rescuer to take additional actions when using an AED:

- The victim has a hairy chest.
- The victim is immersed in water or water is covering the victim's chest.
- The victim has an implanted defibrillator or pacemaker.
- The victim has a transdermal medication patch or other object on the surface of the skin where the AED pads are placed.

Hairy Chest

If a teen or adult victim has a lot of chest hair, the AED pads may not properly stick to the skin on the chest. If this occurs, the AED will not be able to analyze the victim's heart rhythm. The AED will then give a "check electrodes" or "check electrode pads" message.

Step	Action
1	If the pads stick to the hair instead of the skin, press down firmly on each pad.
2	If the AED continues to prompt you to "check pads" or "check electrodes," quickly pull off the pads. This will remove a large amount of hair and should allow the pads to stick to the skin.
3	If a large amount of hair still remains where you will put the pads, shave the area with the razor in the AED carrying case.
4	Put on a new set of pads. Follow the AED voice prompts.

Water

Water is a good conductor of electricity. Do not use an AED in water. If the victim is in water, pull the victim out of the water. If the victim is lying in water or the chest is covered with water, the water may conduct the shock electricity across the skin of the victim's chest. This prevents the delivery of an adequate shock dose to the heart. If water is covering the victim's chest, quickly wipe the chest before attaching the AED pads.

If the victim is lying on snow or in a small puddle, you may use the AED.

Implanted Defibrillators and Pacemakers

Victims with a high risk for sudden cardiac arrest may have implanted defibrillators/pacemakers that automatically deliver shocks directly to the heart. You can immediately identify these devices because they create a hard lump beneath the skin of the upper chest or abdomen. The lump is half the size of a deck of cards, with an overlying scar. If you place an AED pad directly over an implanted medical device, the device may block delivery of the shock to the heart.

If you identify an implanted defibrillator/pacemaker:

- If possible, avoid placing the AED pad directly over the implanted device.
- Follow the normal steps for operating an AED.

Occasionally the analysis and shock cycles of implanted defibrillators and AEDs will conflict. If the implanted defibrillator is delivering shocks to the victim (the victim's muscles contract in a manner like that observed after an AED shock), allow 30 to 60 seconds for the implanted defibrillator to complete the treatment cycle before delivering a shock from the AED.

Transdermal Medication Patches

Do not place AED pads directly on top of a medication patch (eg, a patch of nitroglycerin, nicotine, pain medication, hormone replacement therapy, or antihypertensive medication). The medication patch may block the transfer of energy from the AED pad to the heart and may cause small burns to the skin.

If it won't delay shock delivery, remove the patch and wipe the area clean before attaching the AED pad.

2-Rescuer BLS Sequence With an AED

2 Rescuers With an AED

Follow these BLS steps for 2 rescuers with an AED:

Step	Action
1	**Check for response and check breathing:** If the victim does not respond and is not breathing or not breathing normally (ie, only gasping): • The first rescuer stays with the victim and performs the next steps until the second rescuer returns with the AED. • The second rescuer activates the emergency response system and gets the AED.
2	**Check for pulse:** If a pulse is not definitely felt in 10 seconds: • The first rescuer removes or moves clothing covering the victim's chest (this will allow rescuers to apply the AED pads when the AED arrives). • The first rescuer starts CPR, beginning with chest compressions.
3	**Attempt defibrillation with the AED:** • When the AED arrives, place it at the victim's side near the rescuer who will be operating it. The AED is usually placed on the side of the victim opposite the rescuer who is performing chest compressions (Figure 16).
4	**POWER ON the AED** (the AED will then guide you through the next steps) (Figure 17). • Open the carrying case or the top of the AED. • Turn the power on (some devices will "power on" automatically when you open the lid or case).

5	**ATTACH** AED pads to the victim's bare chest (Figure 18).
	
	• Choose adult pads (not child pads or a child system) for victims 8 years of age and older.
	• Peel the backing away from the AED pads.
	• Attach the adhesive AED pads to the victim's bare chest.
	    – Place one AED pad on the victim's upper-right chest (directly below the collarbone).
	    – Place the other pad to the side of the left nipple, with the top edge of the pad a few inches below the armpit (Figure 15).
	• Attach the AED connecting cables to the AED box (some are preconnected).

6	"Clear" the victim and **ANALYZE** the rhythm (Figure 19). • If the AED prompts you, clear the victim during analysis. Be sure no one is touching the victim, not even the rescuer in charge of giving breaths. • Some AEDs will tell you to push a button to allow the AED to begin analyzing the heart rhythm; others will do that automatically. The AED may take about 5 to 15 seconds to analyze. • The AED then tells you if a shock is needed.

(continued)

(continued)

Step	Action
7	**If the AED advises a shock, it will tell you to clear the victim.** • Clear the victim before delivering the shock (Figure 20A): be sure no one is touching the victim. • Loudly state a "clear the victim" message, such as "Everybody clear" or simply "Clear." • Look to be sure no one is in contact with the victim. • Press the **SHOCK** button (Figure 20B). • The shock will produce a sudden contraction of the victim's muscles.
8	If no shock is needed, and after any shock delivery, **immediately resume CPR,** starting with chest compressions (Figure 21).
9	After 5 cycles or about 2 minutes of CPR, the AED will prompt you to repeat steps 6 and 7. If "no shock advised," immediately restart CPR beginning with chest compressions.

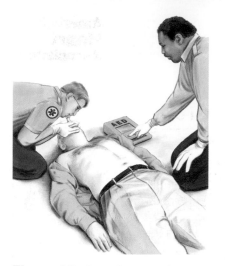

Figure 16. Second rescuer places AED beside victim.

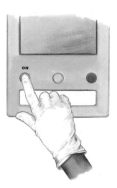

Figure 17. AED operator turns AED on.

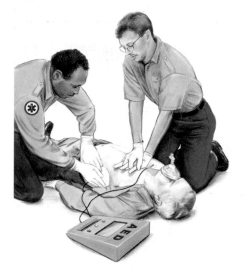

Figure 18. Rescuer attaches AED pads to the victim and then attaches the electrodes to the AED.

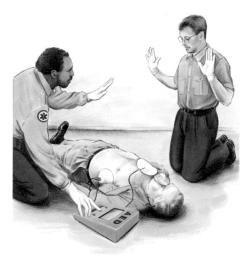

Figure 19. The AED operator clears the victim before rhythm analysis. If needed, the AED operator then activates the ANALYZE feature of the AED.

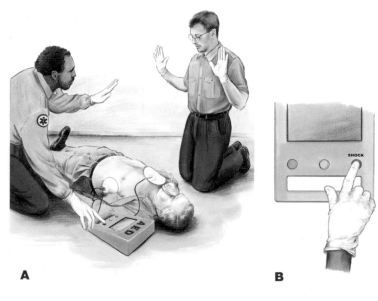

A

B

Figure 20. **A,** The AED operator clears the victim before delivering a shock. **B,** When everyone is clear of the victim, the AED operator presses the SHOCK button.

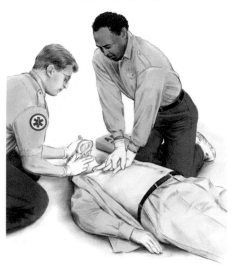

Figure 21. If no shock is indicated and immediately after any shock delivered, rescuers start CPR, beginning with chest compressions (C-A-B sequence).

BLS for Healthcare Providers Course
1- and 2-Rescuer Adult BLS With AED Skills Testing Sheet

See 1- and 2-Rescuer Adult BLS With AED Skills Testing Criteria and Descriptors on next page

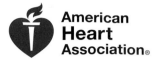
American Heart Association®

Student Name: _____ Test Date: _____

CPR Skills (circle one):	**Pass**	**Needs Remediation**	
AED Skills (circle one):	**Pass**	**Needs Remediation**	

Skill Step	Critical Performance Criteria	✓ if done correctly	
1-Rescuer Adult BLS Skills Evaluation During this first phase, evaluate the first rescuer's ability to initiate BLS and deliver high-quality CPR for 5 cycles.			
1	ASSESSES: Checks for response and for no breathing or no normal breathing, only gasping (at least 5 seconds but no more than 10 seconds)		
2	ACTIVATES emergency response system		
3	Checks for PULSE (no more than 10 seconds)		
4	GIVES HIGH-QUALITY CPR:		
	• Correct compression HAND PLACEMENT	Cycle 1:	
	• ADEQUATE RATE: At least 100/min (ie, delivers each set of 30 chest compressions in 18 seconds or less)	Cycle 2:	Time:
	• ADEQUATE DEPTH: Delivers compressions at least 2 inches in depth (at least 23 out of 30)	Cycle 3:	
	• ALLOWS COMPLETE CHEST RECOIL (at least 23 out of 30)	Cycle 4:	
	• MINIMIZES INTERRUPTIONS: Gives 2 breaths with pocket mask in less than 10 seconds	Cycle 5:	
Second Rescuer AED Skills Evaluation and SWITCH During this next phase, evaluate the second rescuer's ability to use the AED and both rescuers' abilities to switch roles.			
5	DURING FIFTH SET OF COMPRESSIONS: Second rescuer arrives with AED and bag-mask device, turns on AED, and applies pads		
6	First rescuer continues compressions while second rescuer turns on AED and applies pads		
7	Second rescuer clears victim, allowing AED to analyze—RESCUERS SWITCH		
8	If AED indicates a shockable rhythm, second rescuer clears victim again and delivers shock		
First Rescuer Bag-Mask Ventilation During this next phase, evaluate the first rescuer's ability to give breaths with a bag-mask.			
9	Both rescuers RESUME HIGH-QUALITY CPR immediately after shock delivery:	Cycle 1	Cycle 2
	• SECOND RESCUER gives 30 compressions immediately after shock delivery (for 2 cycles)		
	• FIRST RESCUER successfully delivers 2 breaths with bag-mask (for 2 cycles)		
AFTER 2 CYCLES, STOP THE EVALUATION			

- If the student completes all steps successfully (a ✓ in each box to the right of Critical Performance Criteria), the student passed this scenario.
- If the student does not complete all steps successfully (as indicated by a blank box to the right of any of the Critical Performance Criteria), give the form to the student for review as part of the student's remediation.
- After reviewing the form, the student will give the form to the instructor who is reevaluating the student. The student will reperform the entire scenario, and the instructor will notate the reevaluation on this same form.
- If the reevaluation is to be done at a different time, the instructor should collect this sheet before the student leaves the classroom.

	Remediation (if needed):
Instructor Signature: _____	Instructor Signature: _____
Print Instructor Name:_____	Print Instructor Name:_____
Date: _____	Date: _____

BLS for Healthcare Providers Course
1- and 2-Rescuer Adult BLS With AED Skills Testing Criteria and Descriptors

1. **Assesses victim (Steps 1 and 2, assessment and activation, must be completed within 10 seconds of arrival at scene):**
   - Checks for unresponsiveness (this MUST precede starting compressions)
   - Checks for no breathing or no normal breathing (only gasping)

2. **Activates emergency response system (Steps 1 and 2, assessment and activation, must be completed within 10 seconds of arrival at scene):**
   - Shouts for help/directs someone to call for help AND get AED/defibrillator

3. **Checks for pulse:**
   - Checks carotid pulse
   - This should take no more than 10 seconds

4. **Delivers high-quality CPR (initiates compressions within 10 seconds of identifying cardiac arrest):**
   - Correct placement of hands/fingers in center of chest
     - Adult: Lower half of breastbone
     - Adult: 2-handed (second hand on top of the first or grasping the wrist of the first hand)
   - Compression rate of at least 100/min
     - Delivers 30 compressions in 18 seconds or less
   - Adequate depth for age
   - Adult: at least 2 inches (5 cm)
   - Complete chest recoil after each compression
   - Minimizes interruptions in compressions:
     - Less than 10 seconds between last compression of one cycle and first compression of next cycle
     - Compressions not interrupted until AED analyzing rhythm
     - Compressions resumed immediately after shock/no shock indicated

5-8. **Integrates prompt and proper use of AED with CPR:**
   - Turns AED on
   - Places proper-sized pads for victim's age in correct location
   - Clears rescuers from victim for AED to analyze rhythm (pushes ANALYZE button if required by device)
   - Clears victim and delivers shock
   - Resumes chest compressions immediately after shock delivery
   - Does NOT turn off AED during CPR
   - Provides safe environment for rescuers during AED shock delivery:
     - Communicates clearly to all other rescuers to stop touching victim
     - Delivers shock to victim after all rescuers are clear of victim
   - Switches during analysis phase of AED

9. **Provides effective breaths:**
   - Opens airway adequately
   - Delivers each breath over 1 second
   - Delivers breaths that produce visible chest rise
   - Avoids excessive ventilation

BLS/CPR for Children From 1 Year of Age to Puberty

BLS/CPR Basics for Children From 1 Year of Age to Puberty

Overview

This section covers the basic steps of CPR for children from 1 year of age to puberty. Signs of puberty include chest or underarm hair on males and any breast development in females.

Learning Objectives

At the end of this section you will be able to tell the basic steps of CPR for children.

Child BLS

The child BLS sequence and skills are similar to the sequence for adult BLS. The key differences between child and adult BLS are

- **Compression-ventilation ratio for 2-rescuer CPR:** 15:2 ratio for 2-rescuer child CPR
- **Compression depth:** For children, compress at least one third the depth of the chest, approximately 2 inches (5 cm)
- **Compression technique:** May use 1- or 2-handed chest compressions for very small children
- **When to activate the emergency response system:**
  - If you did not witness the arrest and are alone, provide 2 minutes of CPR before leaving the child to activate the emergency response system and get the AED (or defibrillator).
  - If the arrest is sudden and witnessed, leave the child to activate the emergency response system and get the AED (or defibrillator), and then return to the child.

Compression Rate and Ratio for Lone Rescuer

The lone rescuer should use the universal compression-ventilation ratio of 30 compressions to 2 breaths when giving CPR to victims of all ages (except newly born infants). The term *universal* represents a consistent recommended ratio for all lone rescuers for victims of all ages.

1-Handed Chest Compressions

For very small children you may use either 1 or 2 hands for chest compressions. Make sure you compress the chest one third the depth of the chest with each compression.

Foundational Facts

When to Activate the Emergency Response System

Many infants and children are thought to develop respiratory arrest and bradycardia before they develop cardiac arrest. If such children receive prompt CPR before development of cardiac arrest, they have a high survival rate.

If the rescuer leaves a child with respiratory arrest or bradycardia to phone the emergency response system, the child may progress to cardiac arrest, and the chance of survival will be much lower. For this reason, if the lone rescuer finds an unresponsive child who is not breathing or only gasping, the rescuer should provide 5 cycles (about 2 minutes) of CPR before activating the emergency response system.

Foundational Facts

Compression Depth, Adult vs Child

Recommended depth of compressions:

- Adults: AT LEAST 2 inches
- Children: At least one third of the anterior-posterior depth of the chest or APPROXIMATELY 2 inches (5 cm)

1-Rescuer Child BLS Sequence

Follow these steps to perform the 1-rescuer BLS sequence for a child:

Step	Action
1	Check the child for a response and check breathing. If there is no response and no breathing or only gasping, shout for help.
2	If someone responds, send that person to activate the emergency response system and get the AED. *Note:* If the child collapsed suddenly and you are alone, leave the child to activate the emergency response system and get the AED; then return to the child.
3	Check the child's pulse (take at least 5 but no more than 10 seconds). You may try to feel the child's carotid or femoral pulse.
4	If within 10 seconds you don't definitely feel a pulse or if, despite adequate oxygenation and ventilation, the heart rate is <60/min with signs of poor perfusion, perform cycles of compressions and breaths (30:2 ratio), starting with compressions.
5	After 5 cycles, if someone has not already done so, activate the emergency response system and get the AED (or defibrillator). Use the AED as soon as it is available.

Locating the Femoral Artery Pulse

To perform a pulse check in the child, palpate a carotid or femoral pulse. If you do not definitely feel a pulse within 10 seconds, start chest compressions.

Follow these steps to locate the femoral artery pulse:

Step	Action
1	Place 2 fingers in the inner thigh, midway between the hipbone and the pubic bone and just below the crease where the leg meets the abdomen.
2	Feel for a pulse *for at least 5 but no more than 10 seconds*. If you do not definitely feel a pulse, begin CPR, starting with chest compressions (C-A-B sequence).

2-Rescuer Child BLS Sequence

Follow these steps to perform the 2-rescuer BLS sequence for a child (no AED):

Step	Action
1	Check the child for a response and check breathing. If there is no response and no breathing or only gasping, the second rescuer activates the emergency response system
2	Check the child's pulse (take at least 5 but no more than 10 seconds). You may try to feel the child's carotid or femoral pulse.
3	If within 10 seconds you don't definitely feel a pulse or if, despite adequate oxygenation and ventilation, the heart rate is <60/min with signs of poor perfusion, perform cycles of compressions and breaths (30:2 ratio). When the second rescuer arrives, use a compressions-to-breaths ratio of **15:2.**

Child Ventilation With Barrier Devices

Use barrier devices in the same manner as for adults.

To provide bag-mask ventilation, select a bag and mask of appropriate size. The mask must be able to cover the victim's mouth and nose completely without covering the eyes or overlapping the chin. Once you select the bag and mask, perform a head tilt–chin lift to open the victim's airway. Press the mask to the child's face as you lift the child's jaw, making a seal between the child's face and the mask. Connect supplementary oxygen to the mask when available.

Why Breaths Are Important for Infants and Children in Cardiac Arrest

When *sudden* cardiac arrest occurs (ie, typical cardiac arrest in an adult), the oxygen content of the blood is typically normal, so compressions alone may maintain adequate oxygen delivery to the heart and brain for the first few minutes after arrest.

In contrast, infants and children who develop cardiac arrest often have respiratory failure or shock that reduces the oxygen content in the blood even before the onset of arrest. As a result, for most infants and children in cardiac arrest, chest compressions alone are not as effective for delivering oxygen to the heart and brain as the combination of compressions plus breaths. For this reason, it is very important to give both compressions and breaths for infants and children during CPR.

Critical Concepts

High-quality CPR improves a victim's chances of survival. The critical characteristics of high-quality CPR in adults include

- **Start compressions within 10 seconds** of recognition of cardiac arrest.
- **Push hard, push fast:** Compress at a rate of at least 100/min with a depth of at least 2 inches (5 cm) for adults, approximately 2 inches (5 cm) for children, and approximately 1½ inches (4 cm) for infants.
- **Allow complete chest recoil** after each compression.
- **Minimize interruptions** in compressions (try to limit interruptions to <10 seconds).
- **Give effective breaths** that make the chest rise.
- **Avoid excessive ventilation.**

BLS/CPR for Infants

BLS/CPR Basics for Infants

Overview

This section covers the basic steps of CPR for infants.

Learning Objectives

At the end of this section you will be able to

- Tell the basic steps of CPR for infants
- Show the basic steps of CPR for infants

Infant BLS

For the purposes of the BLS sequence described in the Pediatric BLS Algorithm (Figure 22), the term *infant* means infants to 1 year of age (12 months), excluding newly born infants in the delivery room. For BLS for children 1 year and older, see "BLS/CPR for Children From 1 Year of Age to Puberty."

The infant BLS sequence and skills are very similar to those used for child and adult CPR. The key differences for infant BLS are

- **The location of pulse check:** brachial artery in infants
- **Technique of delivering compressions:** 2 fingers for single rescuer and 2 thumb–encircling hands technique for 2 rescuers
- **Compression depth:** at least one third the chest depth, approximately 1½ inches (4 cm)
- **Compression-ventilation rate and ratio for 2 rescuers:** same as for child—15:2 ratio for 2 rescuers
- **When to activate the emergency response system (same as for child):**
  - If you did not witness the arrest and are alone, provide 2 minutes of CPR before leaving the infant to activate the emergency response system and get the AED (or defibrillator).
  - If the arrest is sudden and witnessed, leave the infant to phone 911 and get the AED (or defibrillator), then return to the infant.

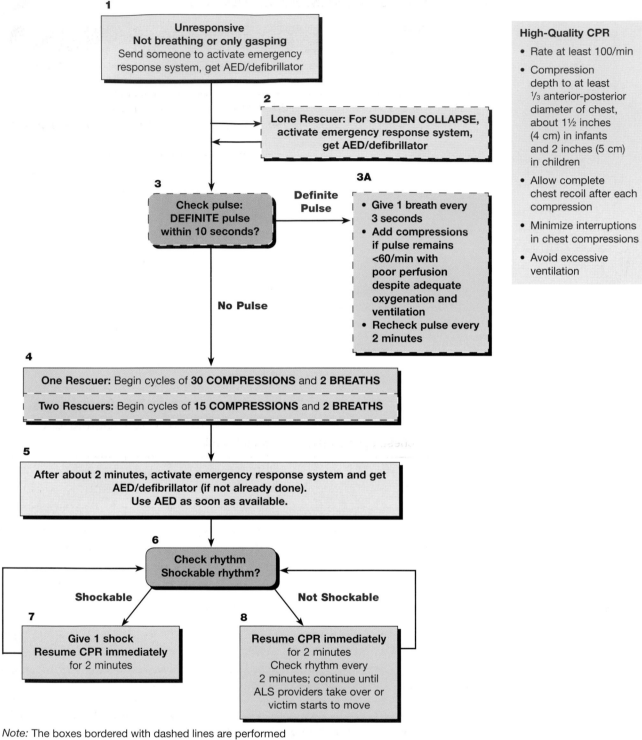

1

Unresponsive
Not breathing or only gasping
Send someone to activate emergency
response system, get AED/defibrillator

2

Lone Rescuer: For SUDDEN COLLAPSE,
activate emergency response system,
get AED/defibrillator

3

Check pulse:
DEFINITE pulse
within 10 seconds?

Definite Pulse →

3A

- **Give 1 breath every 3 seconds**
- **Add compressions if pulse remains <60/min with poor perfusion despite adequate oxygenation and ventilation**
- **Recheck pulse every 2 minutes**

No Pulse

4

One Rescuer: Begin cycles of **30 COMPRESSIONS** and **2 BREATHS**

Two Rescuers: Begin cycles of **15 COMPRESSIONS** and **2 BREATHS**

5

After about 2 minutes, activate emergency response system and get
AED/defibrillator (if not already done).
Use AED as soon as available.

6

Check rhythm
Shockable rhythm?

Shockable — **Not Shockable**

7

Give 1 shock
Resume CPR immediately
for 2 minutes

8

Resume CPR immediately
for 2 minutes
Check rhythm every
2 minutes; continue until
ALS providers take over or
victim starts to move

High-Quality CPR

- Rate at least 100/min
- Compression depth to at least $\frac{1}{3}$ anterior-posterior diameter of chest, about 1½ inches (4 cm) in infants and 2 inches (5 cm) in children
- Allow complete chest recoil after each compression
- Minimize interruptions in chest compressions
- Avoid excessive ventilation

Note: The boxes bordered with dashed lines are performed by healthcare providers and not by lay rescuers

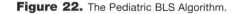

Figure 22. The Pediatric BLS Algorithm.

Locating the
Brachial Artery
Pulse

To perform a pulse check in an infant, palpate a brachial pulse. It can be difficult for healthcare providers to determine the presence or absence of a pulse in any victim, but it can be particularly difficult in an infant.

If an infant is unresponsive and not breathing or only gasping and you do not definitely feel a pulse within 10 seconds, start CPR. It is important that you begin chest compressions if you do not definitely feel a pulse within 10 seconds.

Follow these steps to locate the brachial artery pulse:

Step	Action
1	Place 2 or 3 fingers on the inside of the upper arm, between the infant's elbow and shoulder.
2	Press the index and middle fingers gently on the inside of the upper arm for *at least 5 but no more than 10 seconds* when attempting to feel the pulse (Figure 23).

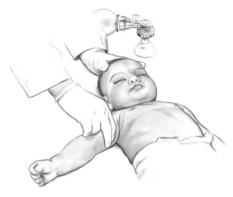

Figure 23. Palpation of the central pulse in an infant; finding the brachial artery.

Compression Depth in Infants

In infants, the recommended compression depth is at least one third of the anterior-posterior depth of the infant's chest, or approximately 1½ inches (4 cm). This is different from compression depth for both adults (at least 2 inches) and children (at least one third the depth of the chest, approximately 2 inches [5 cm]).

1-Rescuer Infant CPR

Compression Rate and Ratio for Lone Rescuer

The lone rescuer should use the universal compression-ventilation ratio of 30 compressions to 2 breaths when giving CPR to victims of all ages. The term *universal* represents an attempt to develop a consistent ratio for lone rescuers.

1-Rescuer Infant BLS Sequence

Follow these steps to perform 1-rescuer BLS for an infant:

Step	Action
1	Check the infant for a response and check breathing. If there is no response and no breathing or only gasping, shout for help.
2	If someone responds, send that person to activate the emergency response system and get the AED (or defibrillator).
3	Check the infant's brachial pulse (take at least 5 but no more than 10 seconds).
4	If there is no pulse or if, despite adequate oxygenation and ventilation, the heart rate is <60/min with signs of poor perfusion, perform cycles of compressions and breaths (30:2 ratio), starting with compressions.
5	After 5 cycles, if someone has not already done so, activate the emergency response system and get the AED (or defibrillator).

2-Finger Chest Compression Technique

Follow these steps to give chest compressions to an infant using the 2-finger technique:

Step	Action
1	Place the infant on a firm, flat surface.
2	Place 2 fingers in the center of the infant's chest just below the nipple line. Do not press on the bottom of the breastbone (Figure 24).
3	Push hard and fast. To give chest compressions, press the infant's breastbone down at least one third the depth of the chest (approximately 1½ inches [4 cm]). Deliver compressions in a smooth fashion at a rate of at least 100/min.
4	At the end of each compression, make sure you allow the chest to recoil (reexpand) completely. Chest recoil allows blood to flow into the heart and is necessary to create blood flow during chest compressions. Incomplete chest recoil will reduce the blood flow created by chest compressions. Chest compression and chest recoil/relaxation times should be approximately equal.
5	Minimize interruptions in chest compressions.

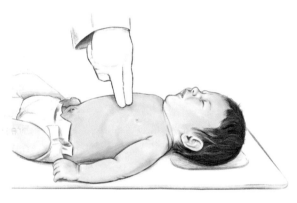

Figure 24. Two-finger chest compression technique in infant.

Infant Ventilation With Barrier Devices

Use barrier devices in the same manner as for adults.

To provide bag-mask ventilation, select a bag and mask of appropriate size. The mask must be able to cover the infant's mouth and nose completely without covering the eyes or overlapping the chin. Once you select the bag and mask, perform a head tilt–chin lift to open the victim's airway. Press the mask to the infant's face as you lift the infant's jaw, making a seal between the infant's face and the mask. Connect supplementary oxygen to the mask when available.

For more information on techniques for giving breaths, refer to the "Infant Mouth-to-Mouth-and-Nose and Mouth-to-Mouth Breathing" section in Part 8.

Why Breaths Are Important for Infants and Children in Cardiac Arrest

When *sudden* cardiac arrest occurs (ie, typical cardiac arrest in an adult), the oxygen content of the blood is typically normal, so compressions alone may maintain adequate oxygen delivery to the heart and brain for the first few minutes after arrest.

In contrast, infants and children who develop cardiac arrest often have respiratory failure or shock that reduces the oxygen content in the blood even before the onset of arrest. As a result, for most infants and children in cardiac arrest, chest compressions alone are not as effective for delivering oxygen to the heart and brain as the combination of compressions plus breaths. For this reason, it is very important to give both compressions and breaths for infants and children during CPR.

Caution **Keep Head in Neutral Position**	If you tilt (extend) an infant's head beyond the neutral (sniffing) position, the infant's airway may become blocked. Maximize airway patency by positioning the infant with the neck in a neutral position so that the external ear canal is level with the top of the infant's shoulder.

2-Rescuer Infant CPR

2 Thumb–Encircling Hands Chest Compression Technique

The 2 thumb–encircling hands technique is the preferred 2-rescuer chest compression technique for healthcare providers who can fit their hands around the infant's chest. This technique produces blood flow by compressing the chest with both the thumbs. The 2 thumb–encircling hands technique produces better blood flow, more consistently results in appropriate depth or force of compression, and may generate higher blood pressures than the 2-finger technique.

Follow these steps to give chest compressions to an infant using the 2 thumb–encircling hands technique:

Step	Action
1	Place both thumbs side by side in the center of the infant's chest on the lower half of the breastbone. The thumbs may overlap in very small infants.
2	Encircle the infant's chest and support the infant's back with the fingers of both hands.
3	With your hands encircling the chest, use both thumbs to depress the breastbone approximately one third the depth of the infant's chest (approximately 1½ inches [4 cm]) (Figure 25).
4	Deliver compressions in a smooth fashion at a rate of at least 100/min.
5	After each compression, completely release the pressure on the breastbone and allow the chest to recoil completely.
6	After every 15 compressions, pause briefly for the second rescuer to open the airway with a head tilt–chin lift and give 2 breaths. The chest should rise with each breath.
7	Continue compressions and breaths in a ratio of 15:2 (for 2 rescuers), switching roles every 2 minutes to avoid rescuer fatigue.

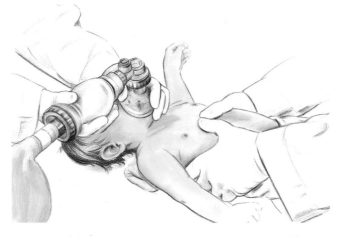

Figure 25. Two thumb–encircling hands technique for infant (2 rescuers).

2-Rescuer Infant BLS Sequence

Follow these steps for 2-rescuer BLS for infants:

Step	Action
1	Check the victim for a response and for breathing.
2	If there is no response and no breathing or only gasping, send the second rescuer to activate the emergency response system and get the AED (or defibrillator).
3	Check the infant's brachial pulse (take at least 5 but no more than 10 seconds).
4	If there is no pulse or if, despite adequate oxygenation and ventilation, the heart rate (pulse) is <60/min with signs of poor perfusion, perform cycles of compressions and breaths (30:2 ratio), starting with compressions. When the second rescuer arrives and can perform CPR, use a compression-ventilation ratio of 15:2.
5	Use the AED (or defibrillator) as soon as it is available.

BLS for Healthcare Providers Course
1- and 2-Rescuer Infant BLS Skills Testing Sheet

See 1- and 2-Rescuer Infant BLS Skills Testing Criteria and Descriptors on next page

♥ American Heart Association®

Student Name: _____ Test Date: _____

1-Rescuer BLS and CPR Skills (circle one):	**Pass**	**Needs Remediation**	
2-Rescuer CPR Skills			
Bag-Mask (circle one):	**Pass**	**Needs Remediation**	
2 Thumb–Encircling Hands (circle one):	**Pass**	**Needs Remediation**	

Skill Step	Critical Performance Criteria	✓ if done correctly	
1-Rescuer Infant BLS Skills Evaluation During this first phase, evaluate the first rescuer's ability to initiate BLS and deliver high-quality CPR for 5 cycles.			
1	ASSESSES: Checks for response and for no breathing or only gasping (at least 5 seconds but no more than 10 seconds)		
2	Sends someone to ACTIVATE emergency response system		
3	Checks for PULSE (no more than 10 seconds)		
4	GIVES HIGH-QUALITY CPR:		
	• Correct compression FINGER PLACEMENT	Cycle 1:	
	• ADEQUATE RATE: At least 100/min (ie, delivers each set of 30 chest compressions in 18 seconds or less)	Cycle 2:	Time:
	• ADEQUATE DEPTH: Delivers compressions at least one third the depth of the chest (approximately 1½ inches [4 cm]) (at least 23 out of 30)	Cycle 3:	
	• ALLOWS COMPLETE CHEST RECOIL (at least 23 out of 30)	Cycle 4:	
	• MINIMIZES INTERRUPTIONS: Gives 2 breaths with pocket mask in less than 10 seconds	Cycle 5:	
2-Rescuer CPR and SWITCH During this next phase, evaluate the FIRST RESCUER'S ability to give breaths with a bag-mask and give compressions by using the 2 thumb–encircling hands technique. Also evaluate both rescuers' abilities to switch roles.			
5	DURING FIFTH SET OF COMPRESSIONS: Second rescuer arrives with bag-mask device. RESCUERS SWITCH ROLES.		
6	Both rescuers RESUME HIGH-QUALITY CPR:	Cycle 1	Cycle 2
	• SECOND RESCUER gives 15 compressions in 9 seconds or less by using 2 thumb–encircling hands technique (for 2 cycles)	X	X
	• FIRST RESCUER successfully delivers 2 breaths with bag-mask (for 2 cycles)		
	AFTER 2 CYCLES, PROMPT RESCUERS TO SWITCH ROLES		
7	Both rescuers RESUME HIGH-QUALITY CPR:	Cycle 1	Cycle 2
	• FIRST RESCUER gives 15 compressions in 9 seconds or less by using 2 thumb–encircling hands technique (for 2 cycles)	Time:	Time:
	• SECOND RESCUER successfully delivers 2 breaths with bag-mask (for 2 cycles)	X	X
	AFTER 2 CYCLES, STOP THE EVALUATION		

- If the student completes all steps successfully (a ✓ in each box to the right of Critical Performance Criteria), the student passed this scenario.
- If the student does not complete all steps successfully (as indicated by a blank box to the right of any of the Critical Performance Criteria), give the form to the student for review as part of the student's remediation.
- After reviewing the form, the student will give the form to the instructor who is reevaluating the student. The student will reperform the entire scenario, and the instructor will notate the reevaluation on this same form.
- If the reevaluation is to be done at a different time, the instructor should collect this sheet before the student leaves the classroom.

	Remediation (if needed):
Instructor Signature: _____	Instructor Signature: _____
Print Instructor Name: _____	Print Instructor Name: _____
Date: _____	Date: _____

BLS for Healthcare Providers Course
1- and 2-Rescuer Infant BLS
Skills Testing Criteria and Descriptors

1. **Assesses victim (Steps 1 and 2, assessment and activation, must be completed within 10 seconds of arrival at scene):**
   - Checks for unresponsiveness (this MUST precede starting compressions)
   - Checks for no breathing or only gasping

2. **Sends someone to activate emergency response system (Steps 1 and 2, assessment and activation, must be completed within 10 seconds of arrival at scene):**
   - Shouts for help/directs someone to call for help AND get AED/defibrillator
   - If alone, remains with infant to provide 2 minutes of CPR before activating emergency response system

3. **Checks for pulse:**
   - Checks brachial pulse
   - This should take no more than 10 seconds

4. **Delivers high-quality 1-rescuer CPR (initiates compressions within 10 seconds of identifying cardiac arrest):**
   - Correct placement of hands/fingers in center of chest
     - 1 rescuer: 2 fingers just below the nipple line
   - Compression rate of at least 100/min
     - Delivers 30 compressions in 18 seconds or less
   - Adequate depth for age
     - Infant: at least one third the depth of the chest (approximately 1½ inches [4 cm])
   - Complete chest recoil after each compression
   - Appropriate ratio for age and number of rescuers
     - 1 rescuer: 30 compressions to 2 breaths
   - Minimizes interruptions in compressions:
     - Less than 10 seconds between last compression of one cycle and first compression of next cycle

5. **Switches at appropriate intervals as prompted by the instructor (for purposes of this evaluation)**

6. **Provides effective breaths with bag-mask device during 2-rescuer CPR:**
   - Provides effective breaths:
     - Opens airway adequately
     - Delivers each breath over 1 second
     - Delivers breaths that produce visible chest rise
     - Avoids excessive ventilation

7. **Provides high-quality chest compressions during 2-rescuer CPR:**
   - Correct placement of hands/fingers in center of chest
     - 2 rescuers: 2 thumb–encircling hands just below the nipple line
   - Compression rate of at least 100/min
     - Delivers 15 compressions in 9 seconds or less
   - Adequate depth for age
     - Infant: at least on third the depth of the chest (approximately 1½ inches [4 cm])
   - Complete chest recoil after each compression
   - Appropriate ratio for age and number of rescuers
     - 2 rescuers: 15 compressions to 2 breaths
   - Minimizes interruptions in compressions:
     - Less than 10 seconds between last compression of one cycle and first compression of next cycle

Automated External Defibrillator for Infants and for Children From 1 to 8 Years of Age

Automated External Defibrillator for Infants and for Children From 1 to 8 Years of Age

Overview	There are a few special considerations when using an AED on an infant or child from 1 to 8 years of age.
Learning Objectives	At the end of this section you will be able to • Choose the correct size AED pads for an infant or child younger than 8 years of age • Tell when to attach and use an AED on an infant or child younger than 8 years of age
Choosing the AED Pads or AED Child System	Some AEDs have been modified to deliver different shock doses: one shock dose for adults and one for children. If you use a pediatric-capable AED, there are features that allow it to deliver a child-appropriate shock. The method used to choose the shock dose for a child differs based on the type of AED you are using. If your AED includes a smaller size pad designed for children, use it. If not, use the standard pads, making sure they do not touch or overlap. The important thing is to be familiar with the AED you will be using, if possible, before you need to use it. When you are using an AED, remember to turn it on first and follow the prompts as it leads you through the rest of the steps.
Use of an AED for Infants and Children	As in adults, use the AED as soon as it is available. Use child pads and a child system, if available, for infants and for children less than 8 years of age.
Use of an AED for Infants	For infants, a manual defibrillator is preferred to an AED for defibrillation. If a manual defibrillator is not available, an AED equipped with a pediatric dose attenuator is preferred. If neither is available, you may use an AED without a pediatric dose attenuator.

Use of Adult Dose Is Better Than No Attempt at Defibrillation

If you are using an AED for an infant or for a child younger than 8 years of age and the AED does not have child pads or a child key or switch, you may use the adult pads and deliver the adult dose. Place the pads so that they do not touch each other.

Victims 8 Years of Age and Older	Victims Younger Than 8 Years of Age
• Use the AED as soon as it is available. • Use only adult pads (Figure 26). (Do NOT use child pads or a child key or child switch for victims 8 years of age and older.)	• Use the AED as soon as it is available. • Use child pads (Figure 27) if available. If you do not have child pads, you may use adult pads. Place the pads so that they do not touch each other. • If the AED has a key or switch that will deliver a child shock dose, turn the key or switch.

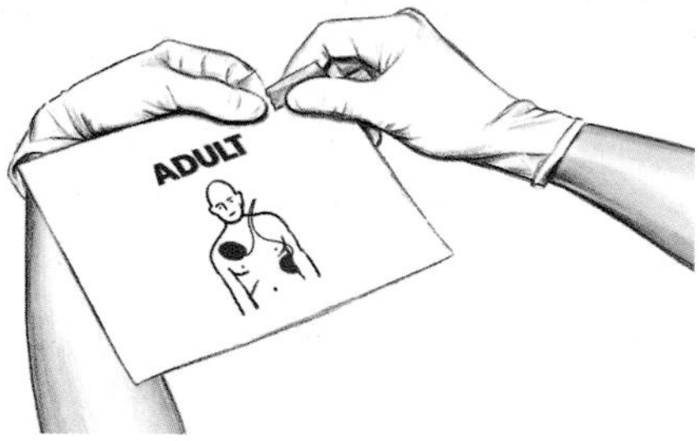

Figure 26. Adult pad package.

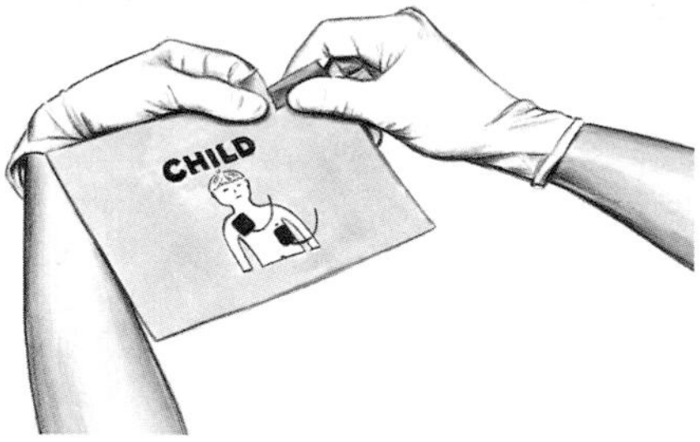

Figure 27. Child pad package.

CPR With an Advanced Airway

CPR With an Advanced Airway

Overview

This section explains how to do CPR with an advanced airway.

Compression Rate and Ratio During 2-Rescuer CPR With and Without an Advanced Airway in Place

The compression rate for 2-rescuer CPR is at least 100/min. Until an advanced airway (eg, laryngeal mask airway, supraglottic, or endotracheal tube) is in place, rescuers must pause compressions to provide breaths.

The following table compares the combination of compressions and ventilations with and without an advanced airway.

Ventilation Technique	Compressions to Breaths (Adult)	Compressions to Breaths (Child and Infant)
No advanced airway (mouth-to-mouth, mouth-to-mask, bag-mask)	• 30 compressions to 2 breaths • Compression rate of at least 100/min	• 15 compressions to 2 breaths • Compression rate of at least 100/min
Advanced airway (endotracheal intubation, laryngeal mask airway, supraglottic)	• Compression rate of at least 100/min without pauses for breaths • 1 breath every 6 to 8 seconds (8 to 10 breaths per minute)	

When an advanced airway is in place during 2-rescuer CPR, do not stop compressions to give breaths. Give 1 breath every 6 to 8 seconds (8 to 10 breaths per minute), without attempting to deliver breaths between compressions. There should be no pause in chest compressions for delivery of breaths.

Mouth-to-Mouth Breaths

Mouth-to-Mouth Breaths

Overview

Because many cardiac arrests happen at home, you may need to give breaths to a family member or close friend when you are not working. This section shows how to give mouth-to-mouth breaths when you do not have a pocket mask or bag-mask.

Learning Objectives

At the end of this section you will be able to show how to give mouth-to-mouth breaths.

Adult Mouth-to-Mouth Breathing

Mouth-to-mouth breathing is a quick, effective way to provide oxygen to the victim. The rescuer's exhaled air contains approximately 17% oxygen and 4% carbon dioxide. This is enough oxygen to meet the victim's needs.

Follow these steps to give mouth-to-mouth breaths to the victim:

Step	Action
1	Hold the victim's airway open with a head tilt–chin lift.
2	Pinch the nose closed with your thumb and index finger (using the hand on the forehead).
3	Take a regular (not deep) breath and seal your lips around the victim's mouth, creating an airtight seal (Figure 28).
4	Give 1 breath (blow for about 1 second). Watch for the chest to rise as you give the breath.
5	If the chest does not rise, repeat the head tilt–chin lift.
6	Give a second breath (blow for about 1 second). Watch for the chest to rise.
7	If you are unable to ventilate the victim after 2 attempts, promptly return to chest compressions.

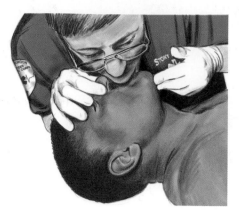

Figure 28. Mouth-to-mouth breaths.

Additional Techniques for Giving Breaths

Caution **Risk of Gastric Inflation**	If you give breaths too quickly or with too much force, air is likely to enter the stomach rather than the lungs. This can cause gastric inflation. Gastric inflation frequently develops during mouth-to-mouth, mouth-to-mask, or bag-mask ventilation. Gastric inflation can result in serious complications, such as vomiting, aspiration, or pneumonia. Rescuers can reduce the risk of gastric inflation by avoiding giving breaths too rapidly, too forcefully, or with too much volume. During CPR, however, gastric inflation may develop even when rescuers give breaths correctly. To reduce the risk of gastric inflation: • Take 1 second to deliver each breath. • Deliver air until you make the victim's chest rise.

Infant Mouth-to-Mouth-and-Nose and Mouth-to-Mouth Breathing

The following table shows different techniques for giving breaths to infants:

Technique for Giving Breaths	Actions
Mouth-to-mouth-and-nose (preferred method)	• Maintain a head tilt–chin lift to keep the airway open. • Place your mouth over the infant's mouth and nose to create an airtight seal (Figure 29). • Blow into the infant's nose and mouth (pausing to inhale between breaths) to make the chest rise with each breath. • If the chest does not rise, repeat the head tilt–chin lift to reopen the airway and try to give a breath that makes the chest rise. It may be necessary to move the infant's head through a range of positions to provide optimal airway patency and effective rescue breaths. When the airway is open, give 2 breaths that make the chest rise. You may need to try a couple of times.

(continued)

(continued)

Technique for Giving Breaths	Actions
Mouth-to-mouth (use this method if you can't cover the nose and mouth with your mouth)	• Maintain a head tilt–chin lift to keep the airway open. • Pinch the victim's nose tightly with thumb and forefinger. • Make a mouth-to-mouth seal. • Provide 2 mouth-to-mouth breaths. Make sure the chest rises with each breath. • If the chest does not rise, repeat the head tilt–chin lift to reopen the airway. It may be necessary to move the infant's head through a range of positions to provide optimal airway patency and effective rescue breaths. When the airway is open, give 2 breaths that make the chest rise.

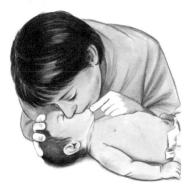

Figure 29. Mouth-to-mouth-and-nose breaths for an infant victim.

Part 9

Rescue Breathing

Adult, Child, and Infant Rescue Breathing

Overview

This section tells how to do rescue breathing for adult, child, and infant victims.

Rescue Breathing

When an adult, child, or infant has a pulse but is not breathing effectively, rescuers should give breaths without chest compressions. This is rescue breathing.

The following table shows guidelines for rescue breathing for adults, children, and infants:

Rescue Breathing for Adults	Rescue Breathing for Infants and Children
• Give 1 breath every 5 to 6 seconds (about 10 to 12 breaths per minute).	• Give 1 breath every 3 to 5 seconds (about 12 to 20 breaths per minute).
• Give each breath in 1 second. • Each breath should result in visible chest rise. • Check the pulse about every 2 minutes.	

Note: In infants and children, if, despite adequate oxygenation and ventilation, the pulse is <60/min with signs of poor perfusion, start CPR.

Foundational Facts

Respiratory Arrest

Respiratory arrest is the absence of respirations (ie, apnea). During both respiratory arrest and inadequate ventilation, the victim has cardiac output (blood flow to the body) detectable as a palpable central pulse. The heart rate may be slow, and cardiac arrest may develop if rescue breathing is not provided.

Healthcare providers should be able to identify respiratory arrest.

When respirations are absent or inadequate, the healthcare provider must immediately open the airway and give breaths to prevent cardiac arrest and hypoxic injury to the brain and other organs.

Relief of Choking

Relief of Choking in Victims 1 Year of Age and Older

Overview

This section covers common causes of choking and actions to relieve choking (foreign-body airway obstruction) in adults and children 1 year of age and older.

Learning Objectives

At the end of this section you will be able to show how to relieve choking in responsive and unresponsive victims 1 year of age and older.

Recognizing Choking in a Responsive Adult or Child

Early recognition of airway obstruction is the key to successful outcome. It is important to distinguish this emergency from fainting, stroke, heart attack, seizure, drug overdose, or other conditions that may cause sudden respiratory distress but require different treatment. The trained observer can often detect signs of choking.

Foreign bodies may cause a range of symptoms from *mild* to *severe* airway obstruction.

Mild Airway Obstruction	Severe Airway Obstruction
Signs:	**Signs:**
• Good air exchange • Can cough forcefully • May wheeze between coughs	• Poor or no air exchange • Weak, ineffective cough or no cough at all • High-pitched noise while inhaling or no noise at all • Increased respiratory difficulty • Possible cyanosis (turning blue) • Unable to speak • Clutching the neck with the thumb and fingers, making the universal choking sign (Figure 30)
Rescuer Actions	**Rescuer Actions**
• As long as good air exchange continues, encourage the victim to continue spontaneous coughing and breathing efforts. • Do not interfere with the victim's own attempts to expel the foreign body, but stay with the victim and monitor his or her condition. • If mild airway obstruction persists, activate the emergency response system.	• Ask the victim if he or she is choking. If the victim nods yes and cannot talk, severe airway obstruction is present and you must try to relieve the obstruction.

The public should use the universal choking sign to indicate the need for help when choking (Figure 30).

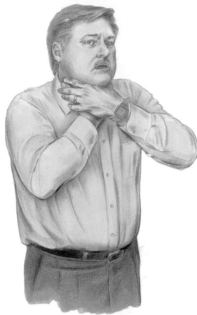

Figure 30. Universal choking sign.

Relieving Choking in a Responsive Victim 1 Year of Age or Older

Use abdominal thrusts (the Heimlich maneuver) to relieve choking in a responsive victim 1 year of age or older. Do not use abdominal thrusts to relieve choking in infants.

Give each individual thrust with the intent of relieving the obstruction. It may be necessary to repeat the thrust several times to clear the airway.

Abdominal Thrusts With Victim Standing or Sitting

Follow these steps to perform abdominal thrusts on a responsive adult or child who is standing or sitting:

Step	Action
1	Stand or kneel behind the victim and wrap your arms around the victim's waist (Figure 31).
2	Make a fist with one hand.
3	Place the thumb side of your fist against the victim's abdomen, in the midline, slightly above the navel and well below the breastbone.
4	Grasp your fist with your other hand and press your fist into the victim's abdomen with a quick, forceful upward thrust.
5	Repeat thrusts until the object is expelled from the airway or the victim becomes unresponsive.
6	Give each new thrust with a separate, distinct movement to relieve the obstruction.

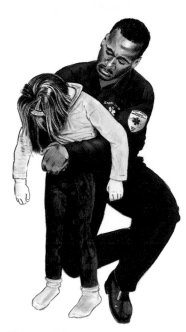

Figure 31. Abdominal thrusts (Heimlich maneuver) with victim standing.

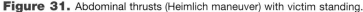

Caution **Pregnant and Obese Victims**	If the victim is pregnant or obese, perform chest thrusts instead of abdominal thrusts.

Relieving Choking in an Unresponsive Victim 1 Year of Age or Older

Choking victims initially may be responsive and then may become unresponsive. In this circumstance you know that choking caused the victim's symptoms, and you know to look for a foreign object in the throat.

If a choking victim becomes unresponsive, activate the emergency response system. Lower the victim to the ground and begin CPR, starting with compressions (do not check for a pulse).

For an adult or child victim, every time you open the airway to give breaths, open the victim's mouth wide and look for the object. If you see an object that can easily be removed, remove it with your fingers. If you do not see an object, keep doing CPR. After about 5 cycles or 2 minutes of CPR, activate the emergency response system if someone has not already done so.

Sometimes the choking victim may be unresponsive when you first encounter him or her. In this circumstance you probably will not know that an airway obstruction exists. Activate the emergency response system and start CPR (C-A-B sequence).

Sequence of Actions After Relief of Choking

You can tell you have successfully removed an airway obstruction in an unresponsive victim if you

- Feel air movement and see the chest rise when you give breaths
- See and remove a foreign body from the victim's mouth

After you relieve choking in an unresponsive victim, treat him or her as you would any unresponsive victim (ie, check response, breathing, and pulse), and provide CPR or rescue breathing as needed. If the victim responds, encourage the victim to seek immediate medical attention to ensure that the victim does not have a complication from abdominal thrusts.

Relief of Choking in Infants

Overview

This section covers the steps to relieve choking (foreign-body airway obstruction) in an infant. For information on relieving choking in a child 1 year of age and older, see "Relief of Choking in Victims 1 Year of Age and Older."

Learning Objectives

At the end of this section you will be able to show how to relieve choking in responsive and unresponsive infants.

Recognizing Choking in a Responsive Infant

Early recognition of airway obstruction is the key to successful outcome. The trained observer can often detect signs of choking.

Foreign bodies may cause a range of symptoms from *mild* to *severe* airway obstruction.

Mild Airway Obstruction	Severe Airway Obstruction
Signs:	**Signs:**
• Good air exchange • Can cough forcefully • May wheeze between coughs	• Poor or no air exchange • Weak, ineffective cough or no cough at all • High-pitched noise while inhaling or no noise at all • Increased respiratory difficulty • Possible cyanosis (turning blue) • Unable to cry
Rescuer Actions	**Rescuer Actions**
• Do not interfere with the infant's own attempts to expel the foreign body, but stay with the victim and monitor his or her condition. • If mild airway obstruction persists, activate the emergency response system.	• If the infant cannot make any sounds or breathe, severe airway obstruction is present and you must try to relieve the obstruction.

Relieving Choking in a Responsive Infant

Clearing an object from an infant's airway requires a combination of back slaps and chest thrusts. Abdominal thrusts are not appropriate.

Follow these steps to relieve choking in a responsive infant:

Step	Action
1	Kneel or sit with the infant in your lap.
2	If it is easy to do, remove clothing from the infant's chest.
3	Hold the infant facedown with the head slightly lower than the chest, resting on your forearm. Support the infant's head and jaw with your hand. Take care to avoid compressing the soft tissues of the infant's throat. Rest your forearm on your lap or thigh to support the infant.
4	Deliver up to 5 back slaps (Figure 32A) forcefully between the infant's shoulder blades, using the heel of your hand. Deliver each slap with sufficient force to attempt to dislodge the foreign body.
5	After delivering up to 5 back slaps, place your free hand on the infant's back, supporting the back of the infant's head with the palm of your hand. The infant will be adequately cradled between your 2 forearms, with the palm of one hand supporting the face and jaw while the palm of the other hand supports the back of the infant's head.
6	Turn the infant as a unit while carefully supporting the head and neck. Hold the infant faceup, with your forearm resting on your thigh. Keep the infant's head lower than the trunk.
7	Provide up to 5 quick downward chest thrusts (Figure 32B) in the middle of the chest over the lower half of the breastbone (same as for chest compressions during CPR). Deliver chest thrusts at a rate of about 1 per second, each with the intention of creating enough force to dislodge the foreign body.
8	Repeat the sequence of up to 5 back slaps and up to 5 chest thrusts until the object is removed or the infant becomes unresponsive.

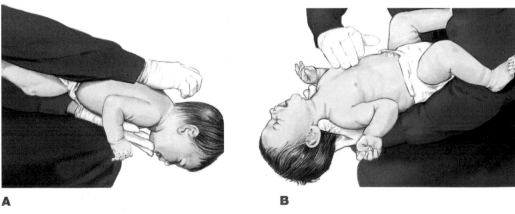

A **B**

Figure 32. Relief of choking in an infant. **A,** Back slaps. **B,** Chest thrusts.

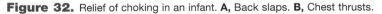

Relieving Choking in an Unresponsive Infant

Do not perform blind finger sweeps in infants and children because sweeps may push the foreign body back into the airway, causing further obstruction or injury.

If the infant victim becomes unresponsive, stop giving back slaps and begin CPR.

To relieve choking in an unresponsive infant, perform the following steps:

Step	Action
1	Call for help. If someone responds, send that person to activate the emergency response system. Place the infant on a firm, flat surface.
2	Begin CPR (starting with compressions) with 1 extra step: each time you open the airway, look for the obstructing object in the back of the throat. If you see an object and can easily remove it, remove it.
3	After approximately 2 minutes of CPR (C-A-B sequence), activate the emergency response system (if no one has done so).

Healthcare Provider Summary of Steps of CPR for Adults, Children, and Infants

Component	Recommendations		
	Adults	**Children**	**Infants**
Recognition	Unresponsive (for all ages)		
	No breathing or no normal breathing (ie, only gasping)	No breathing or only gasping	
	No pulse felt within 10 seconds		
CPR sequence	Chest compressions, Airway, Breathing (C-A-B)		
Compression rate	At least 100/min		
Compression depth	At least 2 inches (5 cm)	At least ⅓ AP diameter About 2 inches (5 cm)	At least ⅓ AP diameter About 1½ inches (4 cm)
Chest wall recoil	Allow complete recoil between compressions Rotate compressors every 2 minutes		
Compression interruptions	Minimize interruptions in chest compressions Attempt to limit interruptions to <10 seconds		
Airway	Head tilt–chin lift (suspected trauma: jaw thrust)		
Compression-ventilation ratio (until advanced airway placed)	30:2 1 or 2 rescuers	30:2 Single rescuer 15:2 2 rescuers	
Ventilations with advanced airway	1 breath every 6-8 seconds (8-10 breaths/min) Asynchronous with chest compressions About 1 second per breath Visible chest rise		
Defibrillation	Attach and use AED as soon as available. Minimize interruptions in chest compressions before and after shock; resume CPR beginning with compressions immediately after each shock.		

Abbreviations: AED, automated external defibrillator; AP, anterior-posterior; CPR, cardiopulmonary resuscitation.

Recommended Reading

Recommended Reading

2010 Handbook of Emergency Cardiovascular Care for Healthcare Providers. Dallas, TX: American Heart Association; 2010.

Field JM, Hazinski MF, Sayre M, et al. Part 1: executive summary: 2010 American Heart Association Guidelines for Cardiopulmonary Resuscitation and Emergency Cardiovascular Care. *Circulation.* 2010;122(suppl 3):S640-S656.

Hazinski MF, Nolan JP, Billi JE, et al. Part 1: executive summary: 2010 International Consensus on Cardiopulmonary Resuscitation and Emergency Cardiovascular Care Science With Treatment Recommendations. *Circulation.* 2010;122(suppl 2):S250-S275.

Highlights of the 2010 American Heart Association Guidelines for Cardiopulmonary Resuscitation and Emergency Cardiovascular Care. Dallas, TX: American Heart Association; 2010. www.heart.org/eccguidelines.

Additional Training Options From the American Heart Association

Congratulations on completing basic life support (BLS) training—an important part of your healthcare career. To advance your emergency cardiovascular care knowledge and skills, the American Heart Association has also developed these courses.

For your BLS renewal training, try these online courses:

In **BLS for Healthcare Providers Online Part 1,** students work through case-based scenarios and get feedback as they move through critical checkpoints.

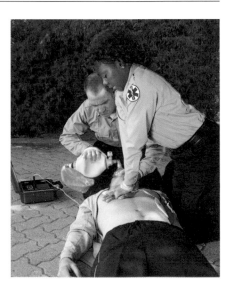

HeartCode® BLS Part 1 uses eSimulation technology so students "virtually treat" sudden cardiac arrest patients and follow interactive, simulated cases for feedback and debriefing.

Part 1 of each course requires 1 to 2 hours to complete, plus additional time for a hands-on skills session.

To learn more or purchase these courses, contact your training center or visit **OnlineAHA.org**.

To advance and specialize your training, consider these courses:

Airway Management allows students to learn, practice, and demonstrate many airway skills used in resuscitation and to increase their awareness of various airway products.

ECG & Pharmacology addresses the electrocardiogram (ECG) and pharmacology, and focuses on specific ECG rhythm recognition skills and drug treatment knowledge.

Pediatric Emergency Assessment, Recognition, and Stabilization (PEARS®) equips students to recognize and begin stabilization of victims before arrest. Students learn pediatric distress signs and symptoms with the use of unique visual cues and tools. The course includes work at learning stations and simulation to see and hear critically ill children.

Advanced Cardiovascular Life Support (ACLS) builds on the foundation of BLS and the importance of high-quality CPR. This advanced course emphasizes effective teamwork, post–cardiac arrest care and integrated systems of care. The course is available as classroom-based or eLearning.

Pediatric Advanced Life Support (PALS) uses a scenario-based, team approach to teach emergency management and treatment of pediatric respiratory and cardiac arrest. The course is available as classroom-based or eLearning.

To learn more or purchase these courses, contact your training center or visit **www.Heart.org/cpr.**

Online

Learn:™ Rhythm Adult introduces students to normal cardiac rhythms and prepares them to recognize basic cardiac arrhythmias. Students focus on improving ECG rhythm recognition.

Learn:™ Rhythm Pediatric introduces normal pediatric cardiac rhythms and prepares students to recognize basic pediatric cardiac arrhythmias in clinical practice. The course includes interactive activities and self-assessments.

Three stroke courses are available for high-level training on the symptoms, identification, diagnosis, management, and treatment of various types of stroke. The online courses offer self-paced, interactive lessons.

- Acute Stroke Online
- Stroke Hospital-Based Care Online
- Stroke Prehospital Care Online

To learn more or purchase online courses, contact your training center or visit **OnlineAHA.org.**

Healthcare Programs From the American Heart Association

The American Heart Association has created a variety of programs and products for the public, healthcare professionals, and legislators that educate and raise awareness about cardiovascular health and disease prevention. Many also provide tools and information to help individuals and groups make an impact on improving survival in their communities. Learn more and get involved today.

Mission: Lifeline®

This national initiative seeks to improve the overall quality of care for ST-segment elevation myocardial infarction (STEMI) patients by improving systems of care. Learn more at **www.Heart.org/MissionLifeline**.

Get With The Guidelines®

This suite of quality-improvement products empowers hospital teams to deliver heart and stroke care consistent with the most up-to-date scientific guidelines. To learn more, visit **www.Heart.org/GetWithTheGuidelines**.